# home workout circuit training

———

*6 week exercise band workout & bodyweight training for fat loss, strength and muscle tone*

*JimsHealthAndMuscle.com*

Visit my blog for more great advice on diet, training, healthy recipes, motivation and more

jimshealthandmuscle.com

Please also "Like" at

Facebook.com/jimshealthandmuscle

And Follow on Twitter

@jimshm #homeworkout

# Preface

H i, I'm Jim, a qualified fitness coach who is very passionate about helping people to reach their fitness potential.

During my time in the "fitness arena" I've been a long distance runner, competing bodybuilder and served a number of years in the British army in an airborne unit (9 para sqn R.E )

You will find out a lot more about me if you visit my website:

## jimshealthandmuscle.com

I'd like to thank you for your purchase and I know that you will get some great weight loss and fitness results if you take on-board and act on the information that you read.

This book will give you many of the tools that you need to turn your life around and become fitter, leaner and healthier.

I have put a great focus on fitness results for the long term in these pages and it is a "no brainer" to me that this approach is the best way to go with any fitness goal.

Before you start this fitness routine, please check out my author pa may be other titles that will help you even more:

## James Atkinson (author page)

Il let you get stuck into the book now but I would just like to let yc if you have any questions or comments, I would be more than you as these subjects are a passion of mine and have been for ma

# Introduction

If this is the first you have heard of me, great! I look forward to our training! This book will no doubt put you on the path to achieving some great fitness and fat loss results. However, this is the second instalment of our fitness journey.

- If you are a total beginner I would advise that you start with the first book as it is a progressive fitness and fat loss workout routine specifically designed for the absolute beginner. The first book is called: *"Home workout for beginners"* and can be found by clicking the link or doing a quick search.

- If you would rather just get stuck into this six week workout routine, that's no problem at all. I have designed the program to be "stand alone" as well as a progression from the previous routine. However, some of the exercises in this book are slightly more advanced and require some form of "base training" before they can be performed correctly.

- If you have already read and completed the first six weeks (home workout for beginners) book, congratulations on finishing your first 6 weeks! This is a big achievement and you will no doubt be seeing the rewards from your hard work.

It's time to step it up a gear and earn even more fitness results!

# Follow along with a video?

If you would like to take things a bit further and get a bit more serious I might have something for you -

Home workouts are great! Following along with the aid of pictures and words can be really rewarding but if you want to take it to the next level, you can follow along with me in real time with the *"Home workout for beginners"* video course!

Yes! We have made a video course based on the first book in this series!

Although the *"Homework out circuit training"* book will give you plenty of information to follow along with and give you the tools to earn great results when it comes to fitness, body toning and weight loss whilst also helping you with the mind-set and prep aspect of fitness that is vital for success, the video course will help you on a much deeper level.

If you are serious about getting real, lasting results when it comes to weight loss and body toning and you really want to change your current fitness situation, then the video course can become your ultimate guide!

All you need to do is tune in and follow along step by step!

In the video course you will have access to:

- **Mind-set Prep and planning** - The foundation of fitness success! This being the mind-set and prep part of any successful fitness endeavour. Overlooked by most people but not by you! The first module in the course will guide you through and help you plan and create your own path to fitness success.

- **At least 6 weeks of progressive exercise** - Let's do this! Starting off with basic resistance sessions using bodyweight, exercise bands and an exercise ball that progresses through the weeks in order to develop body shape, muscle strength and tone and also progressing with these exercise techniques with upgrades to resistance and cardio training.

- **Resistance training and development** - Resistance exercises are upgraded each week to build on each previous week ensuring continued development throughout the training. You will also learn why you are doing what you are doing so when you've finished the training, you will have the knowledge to design your very own workouts and have a great understanding of body mechanics.

- **Cardio training and development** - For the cardio side of the course. We will focus on fat loss and body composition change along with development of our cardio vascular system, resulting in lower resting heart rate, bigger lung capacity, lower body fat percentage and increased stamina. During your cardio sessions, you can choose to follow on a piece of home cardio equipment or with me out in the world. During these sessions I will chat to you about different topics that will further help you reach your health and fitness goals.

- **Downloadable content tools** - There are several downloadable worksheets that can be used in the planning and prep phase along with downloadable material that can be utilised in the 6 week physical training phase to help with tracking, accountability and motivation.

- **How to cook and what to eat** - Diet and nutrition is a big part of any body transformation. To this end, there are several quick and easy meal prep videos that are nutritious and balanced. You can follow along with me in the kitchen or you can take inspiration from these ideas. This is a section of the course that will be continually updated, so more healthy recipes and cooking ideas will pop up as time goes by.

- **Lifetime access** - When you sign up for the course, you will have lifetime access. This means that you can work through the course at your own pace. I actually recommend that if you get to a certain week and the upgrades are a bit tough, that you repeat the week. Although this is advertised as a 6 week long course, it can be completed in 12, 16 or even more weeks. It's important to progress with the exercise choices but consistency is arguably more important.

I could talk a lot more about the benefits of signing up for the video course but I will let you check it out for yourself and if you have any questions, please drop me an email at – Jim@jimshealthandmuscle.com

You can check this video course out by heading over to Yourfitnesssuccess.com for more info.

# Health check

B efore you embark on any fitness routine please consult your Doctor.

- Do not exercise if you are unwell.
- Stop if you feel pain and if the pain does not subside then see your Doctor.
- Do not exercise if you have taken alcohol or had a large meal in the last few hours.
- If you are taking medication please check with your Doctor to make sure it is ok for you to exercise.
- If in doubt at all please check with your Doctor first, you may even want to take this routine and go through it with them. It may be helpful to ask for a blood pressure, cholesterol and weight check. You can then have these read again in a few months after exercise to see the benefit.

# Important! Please read...

———

I am very aware that you probably bought this book hoping that you would just simply follow a step by step fitness routine that would get you some great fitness results. And you will find exactly that here!

However, there is so much more involved in achieving your fitness goals that you have to consider if you truly wish to succeed.

From my experience in this industry and indeed many aspects of life itself, I have noticed that goals, whether they are fitness related or otherwise are often never planned out correctly and this lack of planning ultimately causes the ambition in the plan to quickly waiver and ultimately the plan fails.

This is why I have taken the time to add far more than just a workout plan to this book. If you are serious about getting fitness results, please read all of the pages leading up to the workout plan itself and make sure that you fully understand what you are about to embark on. The more you understand about the routine you are about to commit to before you start, the better.

Please study the layout, the motivation and mentality that you must adopt, take the time to practice the exercise movements and fully embrace the information that is at your disposal. There is so much more to fitness than just working out.

You may find some of the following sections and chapters fairly "information intensive" but I feel that it is all there for good reason. Nothing makes me more disappointed than seeing someone give up on their fitness or weight loss dream in the early stages of their new lifestyle choice. So please contact me if you are struggling or have any questions. I will be more than happy to help where I can.

# What's the plan?

---

Previously we utilised cardio exercise and resistance and used them as separate training entities.

Now this is a great start as you will not only be working towards your fitness goals but your body will be introduced to these different types of exercise.

Another benefit of this is that when your body is trained in a specific way, it will learn to become more efficient in the effect that you are after.

For example; if you jog for 45 minutes at a fat burning pace every day for a year in the hope to "burn fat", your body will be extremely efficient at burning fat after the year is up compared to the first week of this fitness venture.

So now that we have introduced our bodies to basic cardio and resistance training, we are going to "fuse" the two types of training.

This "fusion" is going to be the focus of this book and training plan. This method of training is also known to some as "circuit training"!

# What is circuit training

———

Briefly mentioned in the previous section, I like to think of circuit training as a fusion of cardio and resistance exercises.

Let's quickly jog our memories on the basics of each type of exercise. If you are familiar with this already, good stuff! But I feel that this does warrant a mention:

**Resistance training:** Is usually carried out as part of a routine that utilises weights or resistance bands of some kind in a "sets and reps" method.

For example: If you were to pick up a pair of dumbbells, set yourself up to do some bicep curls and curl these a number of times to target your biceps. The number of times you would curl these is the number of reps (repetitions) in a set.

For general fitness, this number is usually around 12 – 15. You would then have a short rest and perform another 12 – 15 reps. After doing this twice, you will have done 2 sets of 12 -15

You would typically put these dumbbell's down after each set and rest until the next set. The rest period between sets is normally around 30 seconds to one minute. But as the sets and reps of an exercise change from fitness routine to fitness routine, so does the rest time between sets.

**Cardio training:** Is mainly used to work the trainer's cardiovascular system (heart and lungs). Cardio training can be utilised in several different ways, it can be used in short bursts, longer slower sessions or a mixture of both.

Some methods of cardio training include, walking, jogging, running, swimming and cycling. These are all good methods for developing heart and lung function and also great for fat burning.

Circuit training is basically a big cardio session with resistance exercises thrown in...

Or it is a resistance session, but where you would normally rest between your sets, you will be stimulating your cardiovascular system (doing some form of cardio exercise for a short time).

I have designed this circuit training routine to be progressive so it won't be too hard right away, especially if this is a progression from the first instalment of this series for you. So please do not be put off by the thought of "no rest" between sets, it's not as bad as it sounds..... I promise ☺

# Why Circuit training

―――――

There are many reasons to use circuit training as part of your fitness routine. If you are looking to burn fat, develop cardiovascular fitness and tone your muscles, in my opinion and personal experience, circuit training is one of the most effective ways to do this.

If you plan to earn a fit lean body from home using circuit training as your #1 method, you have made a wise choice! Here is why:

**Increased intensity:** Because of the nature of this training method, your body will burn far more calories in a more efficient way than it would if you were to train with resistance only and train with a cardio choice in a separate session.

That said; if you are a total beginner and very out of shape, you may find circuit training a bit too much of a challenge to start with.

**Saves time:** As circuit training is a "fusion" of cardio and resistance training, you will be saving a lot of time cramming the whole lot in to shorter, more intense sessions.

**Added value:** You can always add a huge amount of value in the form of fitness results to these training sessions by small tweaks to the circuits in your workouts. You don't need to worry about doing this right now as I have taken care of it for you in this book. But as you become more experienced in this type of training you will be able to adapt it yourself.

# Do I still need to do cardio?

So, if you are fusing your cardio exercise with your resistance exercise, do you still need to do separate cardio sessions?

Your training sessions will have a 50/50 split of cardio and resistance type exercise. This means that you will be getting a good amount of "fat burning" from these sessions alone.

However, what I would suggest is that you also add a "stand alone" cardio session of some kind to your daily lifestyle. This can be something as simple as a brisk walk for 30 - 45 minutes.

Believe it or not, walking at a slightly elevated rate is in my opinion the most effective type of cardio exercise to burn fat. If you stay consistent, you will no doubt have some good fat loss results within a few short weeks.

If the main focus of your training is to lower your body fat percentage, these cardio sessions should be done at least 4 – 5 times per week and should become a solid part of your daily routine.

Another tip that I have found to accelerate fat loss further is to do these steady state walks before you eat anything, so first thing in the morning. There are a lot of people that will argue with me about this but from my personal experience; this little trick is very effective.

If you are a total beginner to cardiovascular training, you may want to start with a shorter training session than 45 minutes. But it is a good idea to aim for the 45 minute region.

Nothing kills motivation like a "too much too soon" scenario. So if you are just starting out, you may want to start with 20 minute cardio sessions on your first week and add 5 – 10 minutes each week thereafter until you reach 45 minutes.

If walking in the great outdoors is a problem for any reason, you could also use a stationary bike, treadmill or stepper if you have the room at home. If you stick to a steady state type of pace on your "cardio weapon of choice" you will get similar results on either. The important point here is the intensity of your session.

To find the right pace for fat burning, you should increase your speed to the point that your breathing has increased but you can still comfortably hold a conversation. You should also start to sweat. Once you get to this point, you have found your steady state fat burning zone and you should continue at this pace throughout your cardio sessions. In time you will get used to this pace and it will become second nature to achieve.

To help you plan your cardio sessions, you can use a simple chart like this:

## CARDIO SESSIONS

| MON | TUES | WED | THUR | FRI | SAT | SUN |
|-----|------|-----|------|-----|-----|-----|
|     |      |     |      |     |     |     |

FILL IN THE TIME OF cardio session that you plan to do in the blank space below the day that you plan to do it on. Then tick it off once you have completed this session. You can set up several months of progression if you wish.

If you are serious about fitness success, whether it be fat burning, muscle toning, running or bodybuilding, I cannot stress enough how important the planning aspect is.

If you have a solid plan that is written down, it will be easier for you to stick to, it will show you good progression and you will have something to aim for and work towards.

All of these factors will help with the mental game that is fitness and I will tell you that mental robustness plays a bigger part in the fitness/ weight loss arena than most people think.

# Split training

---

Split training is a great progression to all over body workouts and I personally like to plan my routines using this method.

All over body workouts are great! But if you start to train the same muscles with a high intensity, day after day, you will eventually burn yourself out and you run the risk of causing injury.

Although training hard consistently is a sure fire way to get the body that you want, you also need to make sure that you get enough rest between workouts.

Split training will really help you with this. The idea behind split training is that you train 50% of your muscle groups on your first training session of the week and then you train the other 50% of your muscle groups on your second training day of that week.

For example: On Monday's training session, you use exercises that target your chest, back triceps and hamstrings.

On Tuesday's training session you use exercises that target your biceps, shoulders quads and abs.

This way, the muscles that got worked out on your first training day this week will have an easier ride on your second training day.

In this six week circuit training routine, you will experience split training. This is a great way to progress through any training method, not just circuit training.

# The structure

———

It is always good to familiarise yourself with the structure of any new training routine before you start. So here is an outline and some points to note about this six week progression.

In your first two weeks:

- Rather than using sets and reps per exercise, we are going to be using timed slots.
- We will be alternating between resistance exercises and cardio exercises
- Once you start the first exercise in the circuit, you do not rest until you have completed the last exercise.
- Once you have completed the last exercise, you rest for one minute only before starting the circuit again from the beginning.
- Your first two weeks will see you doing: Three training sessions per week with 3 circuits in each training session.
- These circuits will focus on cardio vascular development and target every muscle group in the body.
- Each circuit will be done three times in each session. So that's basically only nine sets per week..... Easy right? ☺
- On the second week, the time per exercise increases slightly. This is to ensure development but also keep the intensity curve comfortable.

From your third week onwards, you will be doing a split routine:

- We will still be using timed exercise slots and alternating between resistance and cardio exercises. And the structure will remain the same
- The training will increase to four training sessions per week, there will be "training session A" and "training session B". Each will be done twice per week alternately.
- "Training session A" targets 50% of the body's muscle groups and

training session B targets the other 50% of the body's muscle groups.

- The training time slots will increase as the weeks go by
- The exercise choices will also become more difficult as the weeks go by.

This is the basic structure of the six week training routine. Understanding this progression will help you prepare mentally for each week's progression and upgrades.

# How to get the most out of this training

Now that you know the structure of the training and that you will be doing resistance and cardiovascular training as a fusion in this routine, there are some factors that you can change and some that have to be kept consistent throughout the circuit.

## Cardio

THE CARDIO SECTION of this workout is aimed at working your cardiovascular system (heart and lungs) and it is also responsible for fat burning. For the sake of this home workout exercise routine it would benefit you to have the outlook that: the more intense your cardio is for the short bursts that you will be doing, the more fitness benefits you will receive.

First let's look at the "tempo" of the cardio training that you will be doing before each resistance exercise in your circuit.

If you look at the training plan for week one, you will notice that the cardiovascular exercise of choice is "Step ups".

Step ups are performed like this:

**Start position:** Position an exercise step on the floor in front of you, or use an actual step, such as the first step on a flight of stairs. Or you can even use a sturdy exercise bench. (The higher the step, the more intensive the exercise)

**Movement:** Stand in front of your step of choice and place one foot onto the step followed by the other foot. Once standing on the step, place the first foot that stepped onto the step back onto the floor, then step off with your other foot to return to the starting position.

Make sure that you perform this exercise at a tempo that you are comfortable with but is still challenging for you. You should also keep this tempo consistent for the full time slot on your training plan.

At this point I really want to stress how important the tempo and consistency of your cardio exercise is. If you decide that you will do one single step up when it comes to your cardio slot, this will not benefit you at all.

It is also hugely detrimental to your fitness results if you "cruise" through, or just go through the motions of the exercise. If you only do as few step ups in your cardio slot between resistance exercises you won't see any benefit.

On the flip side of the coin it is also important that you do not burn yourself out and sprint until you can't breathe in these short cardio slots.

It may take you a few goes at the routine before you find your own personal tempo that is challenging but comfortable. Everyone who attempts a training routine like this is at a different fitness level and most people will start at a different tempo.

As the weeks go by, you will become fitter and you will be able to up the pace slightly. It is a good idea to be aware of this and always try and push yourself. You will no doubt get this wrong from time to time but it is always good to know where your limits are.

If you keep challenging yourself, you will be able to progress to a faster tempo, maybe even reach a sprint pace on these cardio sessions.

Probably the most important take away from the whole "finding your tempo" thing is that you should always challenge yourself because if you are not doing so, you will be short changing yourself when it comes to your fitness results.

These exercise sessions only last a set amount of time and this time frame is very short when it comes to fitness sessions. So whether you just cruise through or challenge yourself, it will take the same amount of time. You may as well make each sessions count!

# Resistance

WHEN IT COMES TO THE resistance part of your training, you need to have a slightly different approach.

Keep in mind that the resistance exercises are in place to target specific muscle groups in order to tone and strengthen.

This is the part where I drone on about "correct form" or "execution" of the exercise. Yes I do mention this in most of my books and many of my blog posts, but I truly believe that this is a major factor in sustainable resistance training.

If you train with incorrect form, you will not only be increasing the chance of injury but you may even train your body to have incorrect posture or even limited range of movement. I have observed people that have done this to themselves and they are not aware of the damage that they have caused.

So please take the time to read the exercise descriptions and study the photographs in the later part of this book. Make it a priority to get this right before attempting a full workout. Practice each one before you start your circuit if necessary.

By making correct exercise form your priority, you will have less chance of injuring yourself during your exercise routine. And if you don't injure yourself, you can always train, so you will always be able to get more fitness results.

Ok, that's my emphasis on correct form out of the way and I am sorry if you are a regular reader and you feel like you are playing a broken record, but this stuff really is important.

In the cardio explanation, we looked at the tempo of the exercise. And put very basically: the faster the tempo or cardio speed that you can consistently keep up, the more benefit that you will get from these short burst cardio sessions. The main focus for the cardio part of the exercise routine is to raise your heart rate.

When it comes to the resistance part of your circuit training, you need to look at it a lot differently. Yes you should have a consistent pace but the exercise tempo should always be slow and controlled.

Each exercise is designed to target and exercise a specific muscle group. The way that the muscle is targeted is the extension and contraction.

For example: If you are performing bicep curls with an exercise band:

**Start position:** Hold a stirrup in each hand, step forward with one foot securing the middle of the band under the rear foot. Keep your palms facing forward and allow your arms to fall naturally at your sides with elbows slightly bent, eyes looking straight ahead and your back flat.

**Movement:** Whilst breathing out, bring your forearms up to as parallel with your upper arm as possible and squeezing your bicep.

You should not rotate your palms inwards, your palms should be facing the front of your shoulder at the top of this movement (Maximum contraction). Breathe in as you return to the starting position.

This completes one rep. You should feel this in your biceps, the front of your upper arm

## Start/Finish Position    Top Of Movement

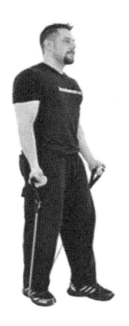 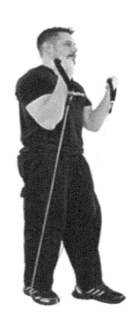

Target muscle group is shown below:

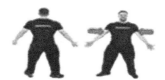

As you can see from this example, you have a start position and a mid-position (Top of movement). Now the key to getting the resistance part right is the movement speed.

You DO NOT want to perform these exercises in short sharp bursts as you would with the cardio side of things.

You should perform these in a steady controlled manner with a count of 2 seconds from the start position to the mid position and another 2 seconds from the mid position back to the start position. This means that each repetition will take 4 seconds to complete.

Once that you have completed a single rep, there should be no break or rest and the next rep should be started immediately.

When performing each resistance exercise, you should aim to fill each allotted time slot for that exercise with a continuous movement of 2 seconds up and 2 seconds down.

## An exception to the rule

LATER ON IN THE ROUTINE, I have added some exercises that I believe can be classed as cardio or resistance. These exercises can also be classed as "Plyometric".

I made the decision to add these kinds of exercises into the resistance slots for a few reasons. The main reason was that I believe these exercise choices to be great for full body muscular conditioning with the added bonus of fat burning.

These are towards the end of the routine so your body has a chance to work up to this kind of exertion if you are not used to it.

Each one of these exercises is marked with a "(P)" on the routine layout page so they are easy to spot. As some of these exercises can be high impact on your joints, you may want to switch them out with another resistance choice if you suffer from weakness in these areas.

When you see an exercise that is marked with the "(P)", you should take the same approach to performing it as you would do to that of a "cardiovascular" exercise (short sharp bursts).

## To sum this up

IF YOU ARE NEW TO THIS, I will admit that there is a lot to take in here and if you have not yet read any of the exercise descriptions; it may not make much sense to you. If this is the case, I would advise that you skip forward and look through the layout of the routines and some of the exercise descriptions, then have another read through this section.

It is definitely worth understanding the difference between cardio and resistance training and the correct way to perform each type of training. If they are done correctly, you will get a whole lot more from your fitness sessions.

When performing your cardio training, you should:

- Train at a consistent rate throughout your allotted time frame for that exercise.
- If possible in short sharp bursts. This should in turn, raise your heart rate
- Always challenge yourself when it comes to the tempo of the exercise.

When performing your resistance exercises, you should:

- Make "Correct form" your priority
- Train with consistency throughout the allotted time frame with a 2 second up, 2 seconds down controlled tempo
- Target and understand the muscle group that you are working

You should also look out for the exercises marked with "(P)". These are plyometric type exercises and can cause high impact on some joints in the body. If you feel any pain or have existing week joints, you should choose another exercise to do instead. I would suggest a resistance exercise that targets your personal weak points.

It is also a good idea to learn how to perform each exercise in your routine for the week that you are about to start before you jump into the training.

# Progression

———

Although this is a six week training plan, it does not necessarily mean that it has to take you six weeks only.

I touched on this in the first book in this series briefly. The reason that I would like to put more emphasis on the progression factor in this book is because some of these workouts will be very challenging to a lot of readers.

With this in mind I would like to add a bit of perspective to this whole routine when looking at your own personal progress through this training.

It is very important to understand that everyone is different. Some people will find this routine easy, and fly through it while others will struggle on week one day one. If you are one of the guys or gals that finds week one easy, great! You can progress to week two in due course.

However, if you really struggle with week one and find it hard to finish the workouts, you should maybe repeat week one so you do two weeks' worth of week one. If you still struggle, just repeat again and so on.

This is a great way to progress with your fitness and keep earning your results. But be careful not to fall into the trap that is your "comfort zone". I have seen this hundreds of times in the gyms that I have worked and trained in. There are so many people that will join a gym and maybe go to that gym three or four days every week, year after year and do the same old routine at every session until instead of challenging their muscles and fitness levels they just end up going through the motions.

This kind of commitment is exactly what you need for fitness success but without progression and more challenges in your workouts, your fitness levels and body composition will not change one bit.

It may sound like I am contradicting myself after stating that you should repeat a week of this routine until you feel that you are ready to move on. This is not the case. It is perfectly fine to repeat a certain week as many times as is needed for you to be able to move on.

However, the more consecutive weeks that you repeat a training progression, the fitter and more able that you will be to progress to the next stage.

I would suggest that if you have repeated the week that you are struggling with three times, you should try the next weeks progression. If you are unable to complete these training sessions, go back to the previous week. You should then attempt to progress every other week until you are able to do the sessions that you struggled with.

This is real fitness progression and it is unfortunately why most people who attempt to lose weight/ get fit or even build muscle never actually reach their goals.

# Rest

It is always a good idea to plan for a rest week. This is a week where you take it easy with training. You may choose to just stay active and just do a walk or some light cardio every day or you may choose to have a total rest from exercise.

Either way this will do you good. It is great to train your body and progress with your fitness goals but it is also vital that you give your body the rest it needs to regenerate and recover. This is why I would always suggest that you have a weeks rest at regular intervals.

My advice here is to take a week out after every six weeks of consecutive training. Not only will this give you the rest that you need but it will also help with the mental side of working on a fitness routine.

# Food

As you may be aware, food plays a very important part in creating your body composition and fuelling your body. With any lifestyle change I believe that if there are many changes going on at the same time, it may cause problems and promote failure to keep on top of these changes.

So as an exercise routine is quiet a large change to incorporate into your life I would advise that you just make yourself aware of the food that you are eating and make small changes here too for now. Remember that a lot of small changes over time will result in a big change in the end.

I will outline some of the ideal ways to cut out bad foods and add good food choices and habits in to your life:

- Cut back on, or cut out fizzy sugary drinks, this includes energy drinks, they are no good at all

- Cut back on chocolate, sweets and deserts. Maybe have one small treat per day

- Eat lean meat (chicken breast, lean beef and fish)

- Eat vegetables and nuts. If you snack a lot, snack on raw veggies such as carrot sticks, celery sticks and almonds instead of doughnuts, cookies and potato chips

- Start to add more whole grains, beans, fruits, and vegetables into your diet

- Cut down on your portion size at each meal

- Don't cut out your favorite cheat foods altogether. Instead, eat smaller portions of this or have this only once per week

So this is a list of things that you can work towards but I would suggest changing one thing at a time and not making all of these changes together. If you are very strong minded and believe that you can make all of these changes all at once and make them stick, great stuff! Do it.

# More motivational quotes

I am a strong believer in the power of motivational quotes and the part that they can play in a successful fitness undertaking.

If this is to be your first six weeks on your path to fitness and weight loss and you skipped my first book, I will bring you up to speed;

In the first instalment, we used a bunch of fitness motivational quotes as a tool for, yes, you guessed it: Staying motivated! ☺

The idea behind this type of motivation can be very powerful. What I suggest is that you print out or if you are reading the paper back version of this book, cut out these quotes and pin them up so they are visible in all aspects of your life.

For example, I use these myself and some of the places that I pin them up are:

- My bedside table so it is the first thing that I see when I wake up
- The inside of my front door. If I am struggling to go and train, there is something to spur me on here
- The bathroom mirror. This reminds me of my goal and I will see it at least twice every day
- Next to my TV. If I am putting off a training session because of the TV, I will be reminded

If you used the motivational quotes from my last book, you may want to change some of them.

If you have dotted these around your house, office or put them on your fridge, after a time, you will stop noticing them as much so you may become "de sensitised" to their effect.

This is a common thing. How many times have you been in a familiar place and noticed a picture hanging on the wall that you haven't seen in a while? It's been there all along, but you are so used to seeing it that it becomes invisible.

Although it may sound corny or silly to do this kind of thing, I do stand by it and can't emphasise enough how much it has helped me out in the past. So as silly as it may sound, it is well worth giving it a go!

These quotes are really a great tool for motivation and in some cases can be the deal breaker when you are feeling particularly negative or you are torn between doing your training or skipping the session.

Don't underestimate the power of this tool!

Here are your quotes to use. Please feel free to ditch these and use your own if they don't strike a chord with you, a quick google search will give you all that you need.

**EVERY TRAINING SESSION COUNTS. SO DON'T MISS ONE!**

**IF YOU NEVER GIVE UP, YOU WON'T BE BEATEN**

## NOTHING THAT'S WORTH HAVING IS EVER EASY TO GET

## IF YOU WANT IT BAD ENOUGH YOU WILL FIND THE TIME

**DON'T WISH FOR IT.
MAKE
IT
HAPPEN!**

---

**WHEN YOU HIT
YOUR GOALS
YOU WILL
INSPIRE OTHERS**

YOUR ACTIONS WILL
MAKE YOU WHAT
YOU ARE

---

YOUR SUCCESS
DEPENDS
ON YOUR ACTIONS

**HAVE YOU DONE YOUR TRAINING TODAY?**

**FINISH WHAT YOU STARTED!**

# Equipment that you will need

It is best to have everything in place before you start this or any other exercise routine for that matter. This is why I suggest that you obtain all of your equipment first.

I know that many people will be pretty anxious to get started with their new routine but I always find that if you get everything in place before jumping right in, you will have a hugely increased chance of sticking to your new routine. After all, this is the #1 reason why people who attempt any fitness or diet plans end up never getting the results that they want.

*"If you fail to plan, you plan to fail"*

So, I would suggest that you set a date right now that will be the first day of your new routine. It's probably best to plan at least one week in advance. This way you will have time to buy any equipment that you may need, sort out your motivational quotes, and familiarise yourself with the exercises that you will be doing and the structure of the routine.

Here is a list of equipment that you will need:

- A set of exercise bands
- An exercise ball/ swiss ball
- An exercise bench/ sturdy chair
- An exercise step or a regular step (flight of stairs)
- A stop watch or phone app that can keep time

Here is a list of things that you should do before you start your routine:

- Plan a start date. You should give yourself at least one week to get mentally prepared. This will help more than you probably think so please follow this advice

- Print/ cut out or make your own motivational quotes and pin them up where you will see them on a regular basis. You should also identify places where you will have the temptation to skip a workout and get a quote or two pinned up here.

- Familiarise yourself with the exercises that you will be doing on the first week. Remember, the training sessions run at a constant pace and if you are pausing between exercises to read how to do a specific movement, you will be de-valuing the whole training system.

- Familiarise yourself and understand the structure of this training system. If you are unsure of any aspect of this, please drop me an email and Il clear it up for you- Jim@JimsHealthAmdMuscle.com

# Before we Start

———

This routine is designed with the whole body in mind. We will be working out every muscle group. Some muscle groups are bigger than others and need a bit more attention so these will be targeted accordingly.

I always feel that it is important to have a balance when it comes to any type of training so this was a major focus of mine when it came to designing this workout routine.

It is not essential that you understand which muscle groups need more stimulation/ intensity than others but it will always help you out a lot more if you do take the time to learn this type of thing. The more you know about your body, the better you will become at this whole game.

However, I would say that it is important that you know which exercises are working which muscle group. This is why I have included a pictorial explanation in each of the exercise descriptions. Please take the time to familiarise yourself with these before your first workout.

## Get set up

BEFORE EACH WORKOUT that you do, it is a good idea to know which exercises you will be doing.

The whole philosophy behind this plan is that you do not rest between exercises and you are working from the first rep of the first exercise until the last rep of the last set.

It is for this reason that you should familiarise yourself with your routine and set up any pieces of exercise equipment that you need for the workout that you are about to do beforehand.

For example on week one, day one, you need your exercise band set up for rows, bicep curls and shoulder press. So if you have the attachments attached to the band and ready to go, it will save you time if you need to set these up "mid workout"

Also for week one, you need your bench/ chair ready for tricep dips and your swiss ball ready for crunches.

It may sound simple to some but it may not have crossed other peoples mind that if you are forced to take these short breaks mid workout to set up or find a piece of exercise equipment because of poor planning, your heart rate will drop and your body temperature will cool down.

Ultimately, you will be sacrificing the fitness results that you should be getting.

Here is a check list for you to go through before you start. Once that you have taken action on, or you can answer yes to the points listed below, you are ready to start:

- Create your own motivational quotes or use the ones in this book and pin them up where you will always see them

- Cut out (or Keep this book handy in your training area) stages 1-6 of your workouts and pin them up somewhere so you can tick the boxes as you finish each workout. It's best to pin these up as if they were a calendar so you only see 1 week at a time. The week you are working on.

- Plan your start date. It is important to have the start date in mind before you just jump in. This will help you mentally prepare.

- Make sure you have all of the equipment that you need

- Read through the exercises and get yourself familiar with them

- Tell people what you are doing and when you are starting. This should give you some extra support and you may even find a training partner to do the whole thing with.

- Do you have an un-interrupted 6 weeks to complete the routine? (No holidays, or other reason to miss training sessions)

- Are you familiar with the structure of the routine?

- Are you familiar with the exercises that you will be doing on your first week? (you can take some time before each new week to do this)
- Do you have a stop watch/ phone app etc. set to count down each stage? (The first week should be set to 20 second countdown)

# Final recap of how the exercise plans work

HERE IS A SAMPLE OF "week 1". I have added some notes to the workout routine that you will see on your first week.

This will help to clear things up a bit further if you are still unsure:

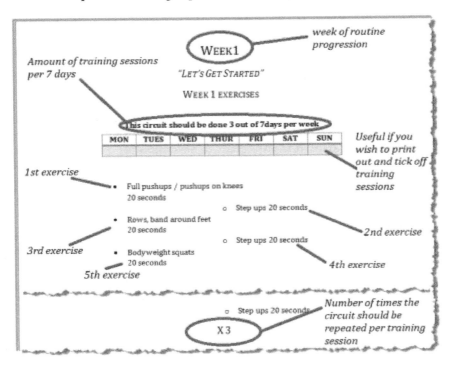

If you are 100% clear on how you will be training, let's get started! Good luck! ☺

# Week1–6 Exercise plan

# Week 1

"Let's Get Started"

Week 1 exercises

**Training days: 3 out of 7days per week**

| MON | TUES | WED | THUR | FRI | SAT | SUN |
|-----|------|-----|------|-----|-----|-----|
|     |      |     |      |     |     |     |

- Full pushups / pushups on knees

20 seconds

- Step ups 20 seconds

- Rows, band around feet

20 seconds

- Step ups 20 seconds

- Bodyweight squats

20 seconds

- Step ups 20 seconds

- Bicep curls with exercise band

20 seconds

- Step ups 20 seconds

- Shoulder press

20 seconds

- Step ups 20 seconds

- Tricep dips feet on floor

20 seconds

- Step ups 20 seconds

- Swiss ball crunches

20 seconds

- Step ups 20 seconds

- Star jumps

20 seconds

- Step ups 20 seconds

# X 3

# Week2

## "Keep it up!"

## Week 2 exercises

### Training days: 3 out of 7 days per week

| MON | TUES | WED | THUR | FRI | SAT | SUN |
|-----|------|-----|------|-----|-----|-----|
|     |      |     |      |     |     |     |

- Full pushups

30 seconds

- Step ups 30 seconds

- Rows, band around feet

30 seconds

- Step ups 30 seconds

- Bodyweight squats

30 seconds

- Step ups 30 seconds

- Bicep curls with exercise band

30 seconds

- Step ups 30 seconds

- Shoulder press

30 seconds

- Step ups 30 seconds

- Tricep dips feet on floor

30 seconds

- Step ups 30 seconds

- Swiss ball crunches

30 seconds

- Step ups 30 seconds

- Star jumps

30 seconds

- Step ups 30 seconds

# X 3

# Week 3

"Getting into routine"

Work out "A" exercises

**Train "A" routine 2 out of 7 days per week**

| MON | TUES | WED | THUR | FRI | SAT | SUN |
|-----|------|-----|------|-----|-----|-----|
|     |      |     |      |     |     |     |

- Full pushups

30 seconds

                                                                - Step ups 40 seconds

- Floor cleans

30 seconds

                                                                - Step ups 40 seconds

- Rows band around feet

30 seconds

                                                                - Step ups 40 seconds

- Bench dips feet on floor

30 seconds

- Step ups 40 seconds

- Double tricep extensions

30 seconds

- Step ups 40 seconds

Star jumps

- Step ups 40 seconds

- Swiss ball crunches

30 seconds

- Step ups 40 seconds

# X 4

# Work out "B" exercises

## Train "B" routine 2 out of 7 days per week

| MON | TUES | WED | THUR | FRI | SAT | SUN |
|-----|------|-----|------|-----|-----|-----|
|     |      |     |      |     |     |     |

- Bicep curls

30 seconds

- Step ups 40 seconds

- Bodyweight squats

30 seconds

- Step ups 40 seconds

- Alternate squat thrusts

30 seconds

- Step ups 40 seconds

- Lateral raises

30 seconds

- Step ups 40 seconds

- Shoulder press

30 seconds

- Step ups 40 seconds

Star jumps

- Step ups 40 seconds

- Calf raises

30 seconds

- Step ups 40 seconds

# X 4

# Week 4

## "Keep it up!"

## Work out "A" exercises

### Train "A" routine 2 out of 7 days per week

| MON | TUES | WED | THUR | FRI | SAT | SUN |
|-----|------|-----|------|-----|-----|-----|
|     |      |     |      |     |     |     |

- Full pushups

30 seconds

  - Alternate squat thrusts 40 seconds

- Floor cleans

30 seconds

  - Alternate squat thrusts 40 seconds

- Rows band around feet

30 seconds

  - Alternate squat thrusts 40 seconds

- Bench dips feet on floor

30 seconds

- Alternate squat thrusts 40 seconds

- Double tricep extensions

30 seconds

- Alternate squat thrusts 40 seconds

Star jumps

- Alternate squat thrusts 40 seconds

- Swiss ball crunches

30 seconds

- Alternate squat thrusts 40 seconds

# X 4

# Work out "B" exercises

## Train "B" routine 2 out of 7 days per week

| MON | TUES | WED | THUR | FRI | SAT | SUN |
|-----|------|-----|------|-----|-----|-----|
|     |      |     |      |     |     |     |

- Bicep curls

30 seconds

- Alternate squat thrusts 40 seconds

- Bodyweight squats

30 seconds

- Alternate squat thrusts 40 seconds

- Lateral raises

30 seconds

- Alternate squat thrusts 40 seconds

- Shoulder press

30 seconds

- Alternate squat thrusts 40 seconds

Star jumps

- Alternate squat thrusts 40 seconds

- Calf raises

30 seconds

- Alternate squat thrusts 40 seconds

# X 4

# Week5

## "Well done! Keep going!"

## Work out "A" exercises

### Train "A" routine 2 out of 7 days per week

| MON | TUES | WED | THUR | FRI | SAT | SUN |
|-----|------|-----|------|-----|-----|-----|
|     |      |     |      |     |     |     |

- Full pushups

40 seconds

- Alternate squat thrusts 40 seconds

- Floor cleans

40 seconds

- Alternate squat thrusts 40 seconds

- Crawling steps

40 seconds

- Alternate squat thrusts 40 seconds

- Rows band around feet

40 seconds

- Alternate squat thrusts 40 seconds

- Elevated bench dips

40 seconds

- Alternate squat thrusts 40 seconds

- Double tricep extensions

40 seconds

- Alternate squat thrusts 40 seconds

- Star jumps

40seconds

- Alternate squat thrusts 40 seconds

- Swiss ball crunches

40 seconds

- Alternate squat thrusts 40 seconds

# X 4

# Work out "B" exercises

## Train "B" routine 2 out of 7 days per week

| MON | TUES | WED | THUR | FRI | SAT | SUN |
|-----|------|-----|------|-----|-----|-----|
|     |      |     |      |     |     |     |

- Bicep curls

40 seconds

- Alternate squat thrusts 40 seconds

- Hammer curls

40 seconds

- Alternate squat thrusts 40 seconds

- Bodyweight squats

40 seconds

- Alternate squat thrusts 40 seconds

- Single leg lunges

40 seconds (each leg)

- Alternate squat thrusts 40 seconds

- Lateral raises

40 seconds

- Alternate squat thrusts 40 seconds

- Shoulder press

40 seconds

- Alternate squat thrusts 40 seconds

- Upright rows

40 seconds

- Alternate squat thrusts 40 seconds

- Squatting star jumps

40 seconds

- Alternate squat thrusts 40 seconds

- Calf raises

30 seconds

- Alternate squat thrusts 40 seconds

# X 4

# Week 6

"Congratulations! 6 week 's of fitness down"

## Work out "A" exercises

### Train "A" routine 2 out of 7 days per week

| MON | TUES | WED | THUR | FRI | SAT | SUN |
|-----|------|-----|------|-----|-----|-----|
|     |      |     |      |     |     |     |

- Elevated pushups

40 seconds

- Squat thrusts 40 seconds

- Floor cleans

40 seconds

- Squat thrusts 40 seconds

- Crawling steps

40 seconds

- Squat thrusts 40 seconds

- Rows band around feet

40 seconds

- Squat thrusts 40 seconds

- Dorsal hyper pulls

40 seconds

- Squat thrusts 40 seconds

- Elevated bench dips

40 seconds

- Squat thrusts 40 seconds

- Close grip pushups

40 seconds

- Squat thrusts 40 seconds

- Military bursts

40 seconds

- Squat thrusts 40 seconds

- Swiss ball crunches

40 seconds

- Squat thrusts 40 seconds

# X 4

# Work out "B" exercises

## Train "B" routine 2 out of 7 days per week

| MON | TUES | WED | THUR | FRI | SAT | SUN |
|-----|------|-----|------|-----|-----|-----|
|     |      |     |      |     |     |     |

- Bicep curls

40 seconds

  - Squat thrusts 40 seconds

- Hammer curls

40 seconds

  - Squat thrusts 40 seconds

- Bodyweight squats

40 seconds

  - Squat thrusts 40 seconds

- Single leg lunges

40 seconds each leg

  - Squat thrusts 40 seconds

- Lateral raises

40 seconds

- Squat thrusts 40 seconds

- Shoulder press

40 seconds

- Squat thrusts 40 seconds

- Military bursts

40 seconds

- Squat thrusts 40 seconds

- Calf raises

40 seconds

- Squat thrusts 40 seconds

# X 4

# Exercise Descriptions

# Pushups on Knees

## Start Position

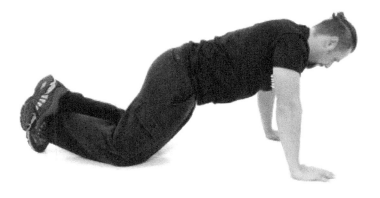

# Pushups on Knees

# Top of movement

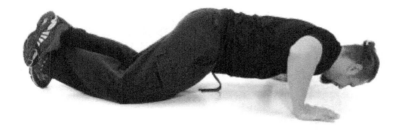

# DESCRIPTION OF EXERCISE

*(Pushups on knees)*

**S**tart position: Get to a position on the floor so you are on your hands and knees.

Your hands should be about shoulder width apart and in line with your face.

**Movement:** Keep your back straight and lower your upper body towards the floor by bending your elbows and breathing in.

Once you're at the bottom of this movement, whilst breathing out raise your upper body back to the starting position. This completes one rep. If you can do more than 30, move to full push ups

# Full Pushups

## Start position

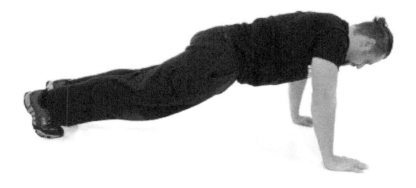

# Full Pushups

## Top of movement

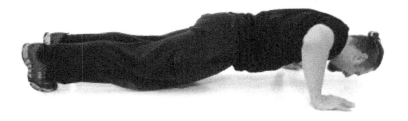

# Description Of Exercise

*(Full Pushups / Elevated pushups)*

**START POSITION:** Get in to a position on the floor so your hands are about shoulder width apart and in line with your mid/ upper chest. You should keep your back flat and take the weight of your body. Make sure that you do not dip your head.

**Movement:** Keep your back straight and lower your upper body towards the floor by bending your elbows whilst breathing in. Once you are at the bottom of this movement, as you breathe out raise your upper body back to the starting position. This completes one rep.

**Note:** For **"elevated pushups"** adopt the same start position but place your hands on a small exercise step. You should perform the exercise in the same way as regular pushups from this position.

# Rows

## exercise band around feet

## Start Position

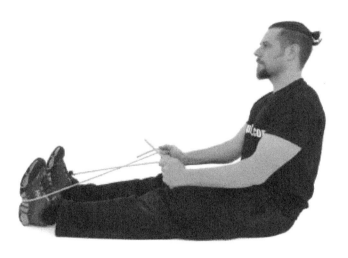

# Rows

## exercise band around feet

## Top of movement

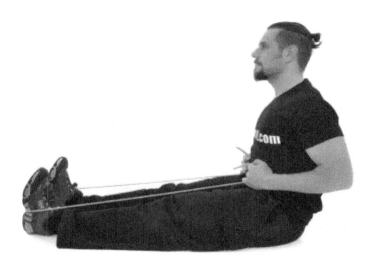

# DESCRIPTION OF EXERCISE

*(Rows, exercise band around feet)*

SELECT AN EXERCISE band that will allow you to perform at a challenging but consistent pace through the full allocated time of the exercise.

**Start position:** Sit on the floor with your legs extended out in front of you. Keep your feet together and wrap your exercise band (no attachments) around them. You should ensure that you have equal lengths of exercise band either side of you.

Take hold of the free ends of the exercise band so it is taught. Note that the closer to your feet that you grip the band, the higher the resistance will be. The more that you do this exercise, the easier it will be to know where to grip for your workload.

Whilst in this sitting position and throughout this exercise, you should keep your back straight and keep looking forward.

**Movement:** Keeping your back straight and torso static, you should pull your fists in to your navel whilst breathing out. During this movement, you should also feel your elbows brush past your lower/ mid torso.

At the top of the movement, you can push your chest forward to gain maximum contraction.

Once at the top of the movement, you should breathe in whilst returning to the start position. This completes one rep.

# Bodyweight squats

## Start position

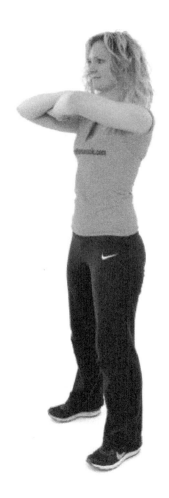

# Bodyweight squats

## Top of movement

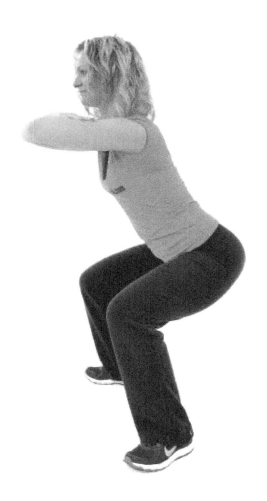

# DESCRIPTION OF EXERCISE

*(Bodyweight squats)*

**START POSITION:** Stand with your feet hip-width apart, toes slightly turned out and your arms across your chest. Focus on a point on a wall or in the distances that is eye level or higher and look at this throughout the movement. This will help you keep your posture and maintain correct form.

**Movement:** Keeping your feet flat on the floor, as you breathe in, bend your knees until your quads (Upper legs) are parallel to the ground. Push back through your heels to return to the starting position whilst breathing out. Ensure that you are always looking straight ahead or slightly up. This will help you keep good posture. This completes one rep.

# Bicep Curls

## Start position

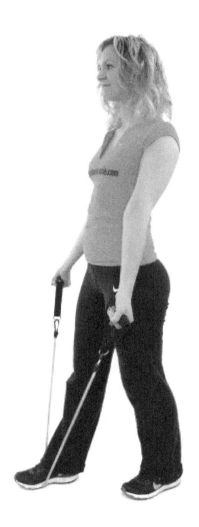

# Bicep Curls

## Top of movement

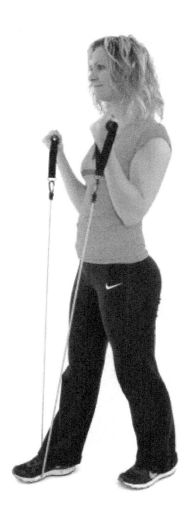

# DESCRIPTION OF EXERCISE

*(Bicep curls)*

ATTACH STIRRUPS TO each end of the band.

**Start position:** Hold a stirrup in each hand, step forward with one foot securing the middle of the band under the rear foot. Keep your palms facing forward and allow your arms to fall naturally at your sides with elbows slightly bent, eyes looking straight and your back flat.

**Movement:** Whilst breathing out, bring your forearms up to as parallel with your upper arm as possible and squeezing your bicep.

You should not rotate your palms inwards, your palms should be facing the front of your shoulder at the top of this movement (Maximum contraction). Breathe in when returning to the starting position.

This completes one rep. You should feel this in your biceps, the front of your upper arm

# Shoulder press

## Start position

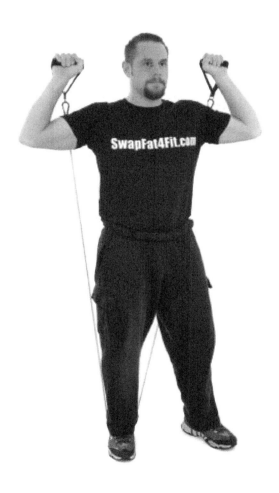

# Shoulder press

# Top of movement

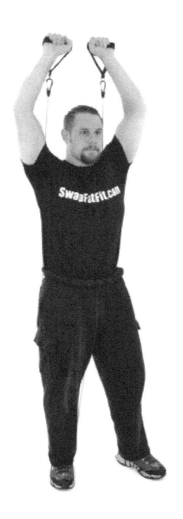

# DESCRIPTION OF EXERCISE

## *(Shoulder press)*

ATTACH STIRRUPS TO each end of the band

**Start position:** Hold a stirrup in each hand, step forward with one foot securing the middle of the band under the rear foot. Keep your palms facing forward and in line with your chin. Your eyes should be looking straight and your back should be flat.

**Movement:** Whilst breathing out and maintaining your posture, push the stirrups above your head as high as you can, bringing the two stirrups together to touch at the top of the movement. You should not let your elbows lock. As you breathe in, lower your arms back to the starting position. This completes one rep.

*\*note; please skip this exercise or check with your doctor if you have a known heart condition.*

# Tricep Dips Feet on Floor

## Start position

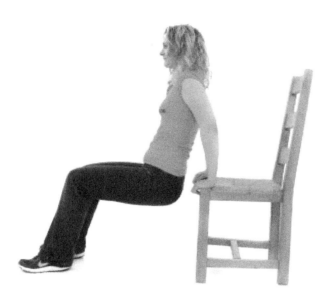

# Tricep Dips Feet on Floor

## Top of movement

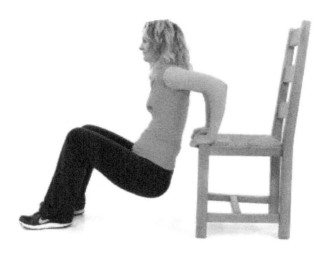

# Description Of Exercise

*(Tricep dips feet on floor)*

**START POSITION:** Sit with your back to a bench or chair and place your hands so that your fingers are pointing forward and taking your bodyweight.

You should now be in a seated position with your feet flat on the floor.

**Movement:** As you breathe in, lower your body allowing your elbows to flare out naturally to the side as you. You should lower yourself only to the point that you feel the stretch on your triceps (Upper rear arms). Once at the bottom of the movement, raise your body back up to the starting position as you breathe out. This completes one rep.

# Swiss ball crunches

## Start position

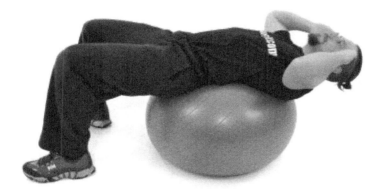

# Swiss ball crunches

## Top of movement

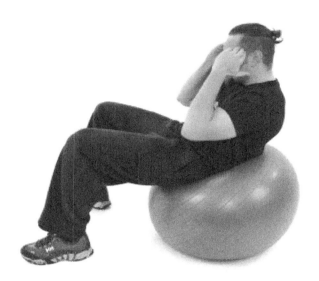

# Description Of Exercise

*(Swiss ball crunches)*

**START POSITION:** Sit on the swiss ball with your feet flat on the ground. Walk your feet forward so the swiss ball rolls up your back and you are in a lying position. The swiss ball should be in your mid to lower back and you should be looking up at the sky.

Place your finger tips on the side of your head.

## DO NOT CLASP YOUR HANDS BEHIND YOUR HEAD

**Movement:** Keeping your feet flat on the floor, you should lift your shoulder blades up, this will put immediate tension on your abdominals. You should breathe out as you do this.

Your lower back should not lose contact with the swiss ball and your eyes should be in line with the sky at a 45 degree angle. Once you reach the top of the movement, lower your shoulders to the starting position as you breathe in. This completes one rep.

# Star jumps (P)

## Stage 1

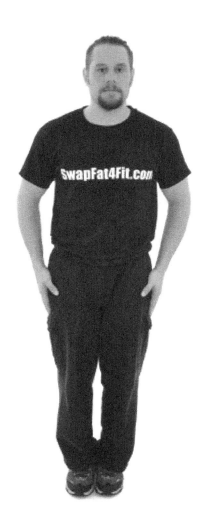

# Star jumps (P)

## Stage 2

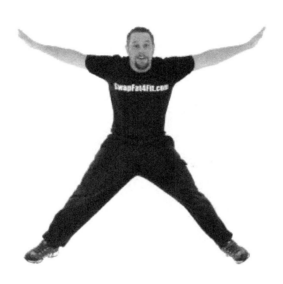

# Description Of Exercise

*(Star jumps)*

**NOTE:** This is a "dynamic" or "Plyometric exercise" which means that it will be done at a fairly fast pace and can be quiet intense. So please keep this in mind on performance.

**Start position:** Stand up straight with your feet and knees together. Your hands and arms should be in contact with your body

**Movement:** As you exhale, Jump into the air raising your arms so they reach at least parallel to the floor whilst simultaneously moving your feet in the same direction.

On landing, your feet and knees should be in the start position along with your hands and arms.

# Floor cleans

## Start position

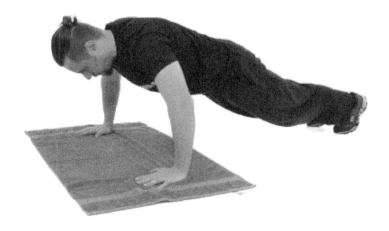

# Floor cleans

## Top of movement

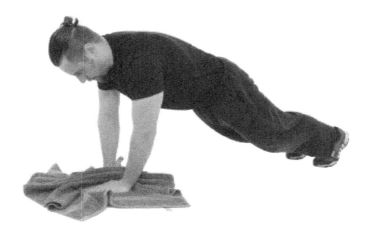

# Description Of Exercise

*(Floor cleans)*

**START POSITION:** Place your towel on to a smooth surface floor (carpet is not recommended). Make sure that is it laid out evenly and to its full length. This will act as a kind of safety feature.

Adopt the push up position with your hands on the towel and slightly pull the towel taught by sliding your hands outwards.

**Movement:** As you breathe out, slide your hands inwards to meet each other. This will bunch up the towel, but your index fingers or thumbs should meet at the mid line of your upper torso in front of you.

Once at the top of this movement, you should inhale and return to the start position. If you got the start position right, the towel will stop you from over correcting when moving back to the start position.

# Pullovers

## Start position

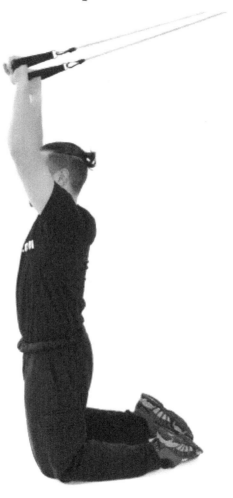

# Pullovers

## Top of movement

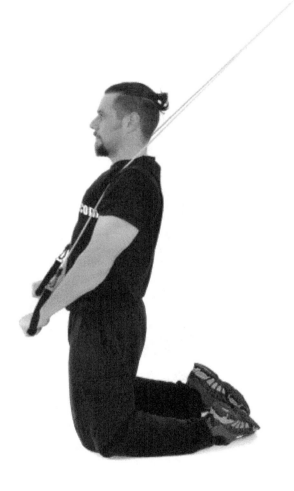

# Description Of Exercise

*(Pullovers)*

THREAD THE DOOR ATTACHMENT through your exercise band of choice and attach the stirrups to each end of this band. Secure the door attachment at the top of a closed door ensuring that the stirrups hang down with equal lengths either side.

**Start position:** Take hold of the stirrups with your palms facing forward and kneel down so your head is at about a 45 degree angle from the top of the door. Your arms should be above your head and the exercise band should be taught. (If the exercise band is slack, try shuffling forward). Your back should be flat and you should keep looking forward.

**Movement:** Keeping your elbows slightly bent and locked in this position, as you exhale bring your palms down until they are in line with your upper thighs. Once at the top of this movement, you should push your chest forward to achieve maximum contraction in your back muscles (Latissimus Dorsi)

On returning to the top of the movement you should inhale and keep your back flat at all times.

# lateral raises

## Start position

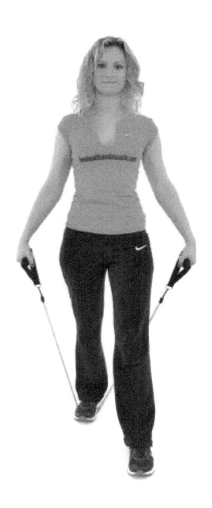

# lateral raises

## Top of movement

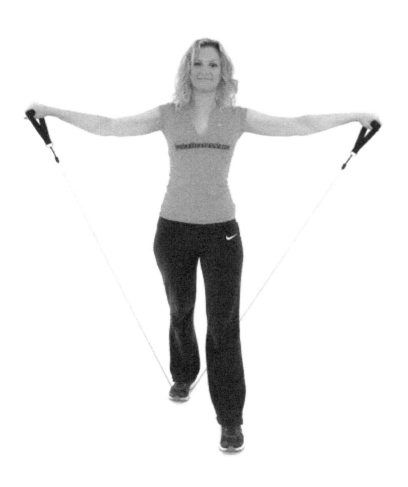

# Description Of Exercise

*(Lateral raises)*

ATTACH STIRRUPS TO each end of the band.

**Start position:** Hold a stirrup in each hand, step forward with one foot securing the middle of the band under the rear foot. Keep your palms facing inwards, your elbows slightly bent and locked, eyes looking straight and your back flat.

**Movement:** Whilst breathing out and keeping your elbows and wrists locked bring your arms parallel or just above parallel to the floor. Breathe in on returning to the start position. This completes one rep. You should feel this in your shoulders.

# Calf raises

## Start position

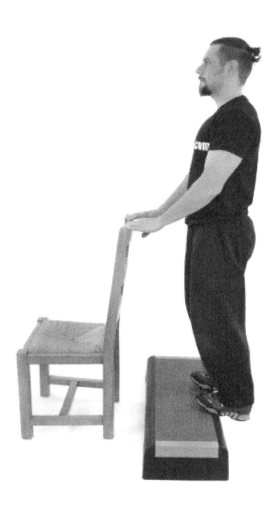

# Calf raises

## Top of movement

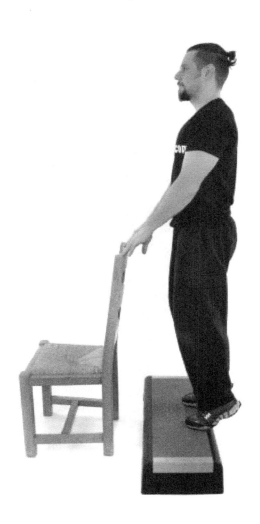

# Description Of Exercise

*(Calf raises)*

THIS EXERCISE CAN BE done by standing directly on the floor or ideally on a regular step or exercise step for maximum range of movement.

**Start position:** Stand on a small step so the balls of your feet are on the edge and your heals are overhanging the step. Let your heels drop down so you feel the stretch on your rear lower leg (calf muscles) ensuring that your heels do not touch the floor. Keep your back straight and look forward.

I would advise that you use a chair or wall to steady yourself. It is important that you do not use this support to bear weight, it is just there to keep you steady.

**Movement:** As you exhale, raise your heels so your bodyweight moves on to the balls of your feet and your toes. You should try to reach your full range of movement so you achieve maximum contraction at the top of this movement.

Once at maximum contraction, as you inhale, you should lower your heels again to the starting position ensuring that you feel the stretch on your calf muscle again. It is a common mistake to not utilize full range of movement on this exercise.

# Squatting star jumps (P)

## Stage 1

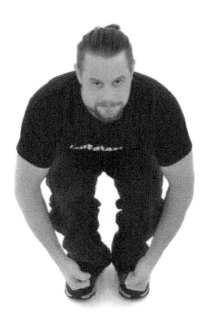

# Squatting star jumps (P)

## Stage 2

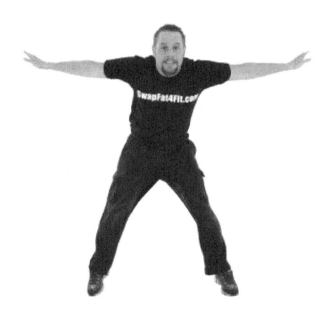

# Description Of Exercise

*(squatting star jumps)*

**NOTE:** This is a "dynamic" or "Plyometric exercise" which means that it will be done at a fairly fast pace and can be quiet intense. So please keep this in mind on performance.

**Start position:** Squat down so that your feet are flat on the floor, your hands should be in front of you, your back should be flat and you should keep your head straight so that you are looking forward at all times.

**Movement:** As you exhale, in one explosive movement, you should transverse from this squatting through a standing position into a star jump ( See "Star jump" exercise description)

Immediately after you touch down, assume the squatting position again and repeat the movement.

This exercise should flow and you should be constantly moving throughout your exercise time slot.

# Alternate squat thrusts (P)

## Stage 1

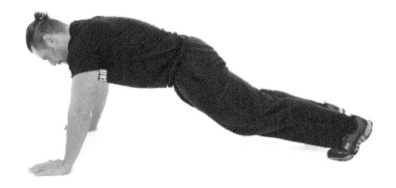

# Alternate squat thrusts (P)

# Stage 2

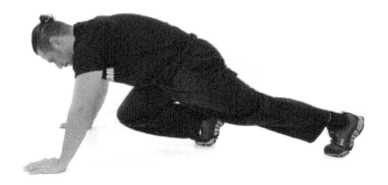

# Alternate squat thrusts (P)

## Stage 3

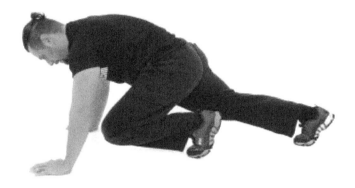

# Description Of Exercise

*(Alternate squat thrusts)*

**NOTE:** This is a "dynamic" or "Plyometric exercise" which means that it will be done at a fairly fast pace and can be quiet intense. So please keep this in mind on performance.

**Start position:** Get in to a position on the floor so your hands are about shoulder width apart and in line with your mid/ upper chest. You should keep your back flat and take the weight of your body. Make sure that you do not dip your head. This is the same starting position as pushups.

**Movement:** Whilst keeping a regular breathing pattern, you should "Shoot" one of your legs up towards your chest while the other stays extended. Almost immediately after the toes of the moving leg hit the floor, in one motion, you should "Shoot" it back to the starting position whilst simultaneously "shooting" the other leg towards your chest.

This exercise should flow and you should be constantly moving throughout your exercise time slot.

# Crawling steps (P)

## Stage 1

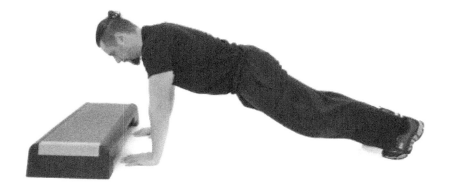

# Crawling steps (P)

## Stage 2

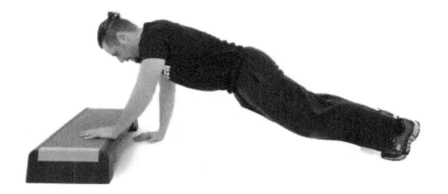

# Crawling steps (P)

## Stage 3

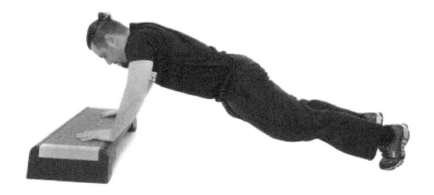

# Description Of Exercise

## *(Crawling steps)*

**START POSITION:** Place an exercise step on the ground. You may want to butt this up against a wall or other solid object as it may shift whilst you are performing the exercise.

In front of this step, get in to a position on the floor so your hands are about shoulder width apart and in line with your mid/ upper chest. You should keep your back flat and take the weight of your body. Make sure that you do not dip your head. This is the same starting position as pushups.

**Movement:** From the start position, place on hand onto the step and as soon as you have taken your body weight with this hand, immediately follow with your other hand. As soon as you have both hands on the step, place your first hand back onto the floor. Immediately follow with your second hand. As soon as you have both hands on the floor, you should start the process again.

It is important to maintain a steady consistent breathing pattern when doing performing this exercise.

This exercise should flow and you should be constantly moving throughout your exercise time slot.

# Elevated bench dips

## Start position

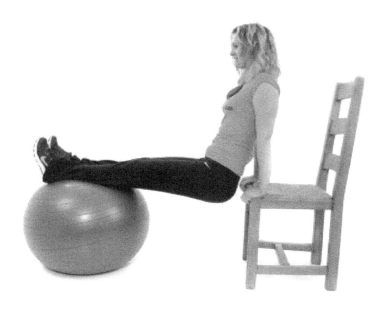

# Elevated bench dips

## Top of movement

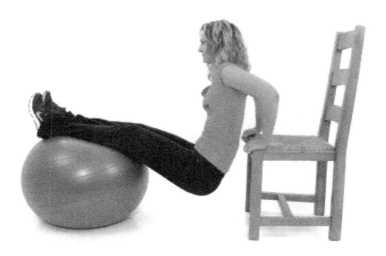

# Description Of Exercise

*(Elevated bench dips)*

**START POSITION:** Sit with your back to a bench or chair and place your hands so that your fingers are pointing forward and taking your bodyweight.

Position another chair, swiss ball or even a step under your feet and take the weight of your body with your arms. Ensure that your elbows are not locked out.

**Movement:** As you breathe in, lower your body allowing your elbows to flare out naturally to the side. You should lower yourself only to the point that you feel the stretch on your triceps (Upper rear arms). Ideally this should be the point that your upper arm is parallel to the floor. Once at the bottom of the movement, raise your body back up to the starting position as you breathe out. This completes one rep.

# Double tricep extensions

## Start position

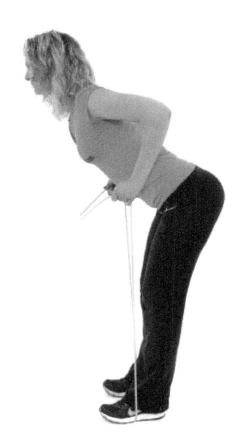

# Double tricep extensions

## Top of movement

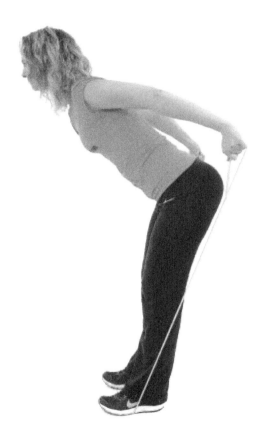

# Description Of Exercise

*(Double tricep extensions)*

SELECT AN EXERCISE band that will challenge you through your working set but do not use any attachments

**Start position:** Place the exercise band on the floor so that it is laid out straight. Stand on the band with both feet so that you leave an equal amount of exercise band either side of you.

Pick up the two ends of the band with each respective hand. Lean forward keeping your back flat and head up and knees slightly bent. Your elbows should be drawn in close to your body and pointing up so that your upper arm is parallel to the ground.

At this point you may have too much slack on your exercise band so if this happens, you should take up a grip of the band closer to your feet. The more tension on the band that you have at the start, the more challenging the exercise will be.

**Movement:** As you exhale, you should bring your lower arms up to as parallel to the ground as you can get them but you should not lock your elbows. It is important that your palms are facing in towards your body throughout this movement and that your upper arm does not drop below parallel with the floor.

Once at the top of this movement you should lower your arms to the start position as you inhale. This completes one rep.

# Dorsal raises

## Start position

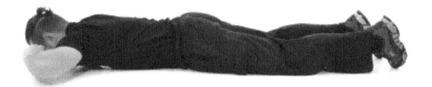

# Dorsal raises

## Top of movement

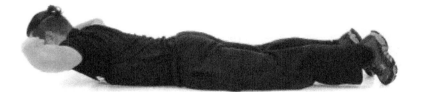

# Description Of Exercise

*(Dorsal raises)*

**START POSITION:** Lay face down on the floor pointing your toes so the tops of your feet are also in contact with the floor. You should then place the tips of your fingers on your temples with your palms facing down and elbows out to your sides. You should keep a flat back and your head and neck should keep this alignment.

**Movement:** As you breathe out bring your upper body off the floor. You should feel your lower back working. If you would like to increase contraction of these muscles, you could also raise your feet slightly simultaneously.

Once at the top of the movement, lower your upper body back to the start position whilst breathing in. This completes one rep. (It is important to remember that this is a small range of movement so don't strain yourself too much at the top of the movement.)

# Hammer curls

## Start position

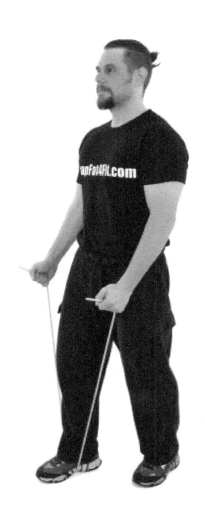

# Hammer curls

## Start position

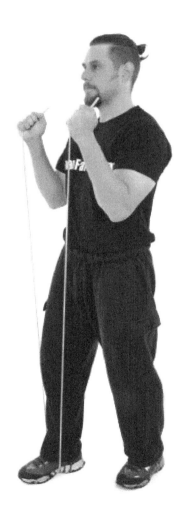

# Description Of Exercise

*(Hammer curls)*

SELECT AN EXERCISE band that will challenge you through your working set but do not use any attachments

**Start position:** Hold one end of the exercise band in each hand, step forward with one foot securing the middle of the band under the rear foot. Make your hands into a fist and turn your palms so that they face inwards. You may need to adjust your grip on the band (The lower the grip on the band, the more challenging the exercise will be).

Allow your arms to fall naturally at your sides with your elbows slightly bent, eyes looking straight and your back flat.

**Movement:** As you exhale, bring your forearms up to as parallel with your upper arm as possible and squeezing your bicep.

Your palms should remain turned inwards for the duration of this exercise. Once you are at the top of the movement, inhale as you return to the starting position.

This completes one rep. You should feel this in your biceps, the front of your upper arm

# Single leg lunges

## Start position

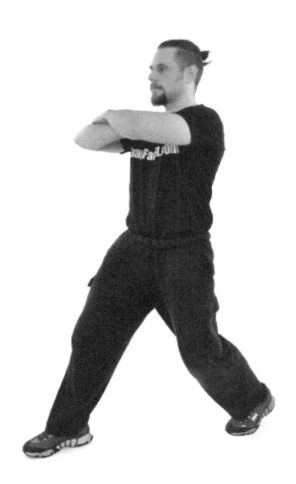

# Single leg lunges

## Top of movement

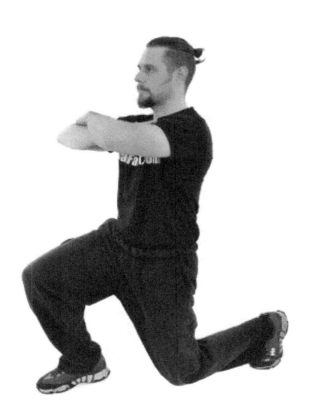

# Description Of Exercise

*(Single leg lunges)*

THIS IS A SINGLE LEG exercise so when your reach this in your circuit training routine, you should perform this exercise for the allocated time on each leg before moving on to the dynamic exercise between exercises.

**Start position:** From a standing position with your feet together you should take a large step forward with one leg. You should step forward to a point that when you lunge down, your leading upper leg forms a right angle with your leading lower leg.

Once you have established this distance, you should stand up keeping your feet planted in this position. Your toes on both feet should be pointing forward and your legs should not move laterally from your hip joint. Because you will have a narrow stance, you should counter balance with your arms if needed. This may be hard at first, but even balancing in this position is developing stabilizer muscles in your body.

**Movement:** From this standing position, keep your back flat, feet planted in the tested position and head looking directly forward. As you inhale, lower yourself down by lunging until your knee is just about to touch the floor, but do not let your knee rest on the ground. Once at the top of this movement return to the start position as you exhale ensuring your feet do not shift.

When you have completed your allocated time slot on this leg, immediately switch legs and repeat for the second leg before moving on to the cardio/ dynamic exercise phase.

# Squat thrusts (P)

## Stage 1

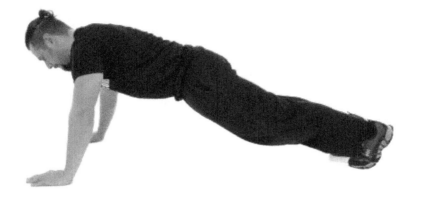

# Squat thrusts (P)

## Stage 2

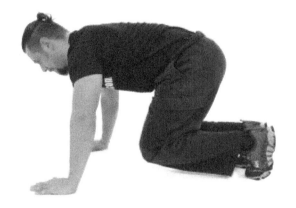

# Description Of Exercise

*(Squat thrusts)*

**NOTE:** This is a "dynamic" or "Plyometric exercise" which means that it will be done at a fairly fast pace and can be quiet intense. So please keep this in mind on performance.

**Start position:** Get in to a position on the floor so your hands are about shoulder width apart and in line with your mid/ upper chest. You should keep your back flat and take the weight of your body. Make sure that you do not dip your head. This is the same starting position as pushups.

**Movement:** Whilst keeping a regular breathing pattern, you should "Shoot" both of your legs simultaneously up so your knees move towards your chest. Your hands should stay planted on the floor and you should not dip your head. Once you are at the top of the movement, you should immediately move back to the start position

This exercise should flow and you should be constantly moving throughout your exercise time slot.

# Frisbee walk aways

## Start position

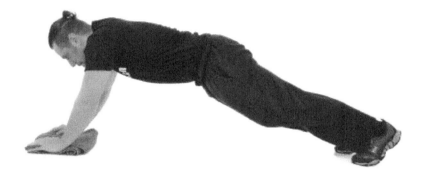

# Frisbee walk aways

## Top of movement

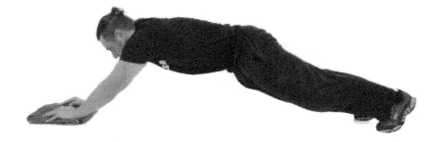

# Description Of Exercise

*(Frisbee walk aways)*

**NOTE:** This is a fairly hard exercise that many people may struggle to perform. If you are un able to complete full reps of this exercise, you should only extend your reach to a comfortable position.

**Start position:** Place a towel on a smooth floor and adopt the pushup position. From here bring your hands in so that your thumbs touch. Your hands should now be directly below your chest.

It will also help if you plant your feet against a wall for extra stability.

**Movement:** As you exhale, slide your hands forward ensuring that you keep your elbows slightly bent but locked in position. Keep your abs tight.

You should only take this movement to the point that you feel comfortable with. The more you do this exercise, the better the range of movement you will get.

When you have reached your movement limit, slide your hands back to the start position as you inhale.

# Military bursts (P)

## Stage 1

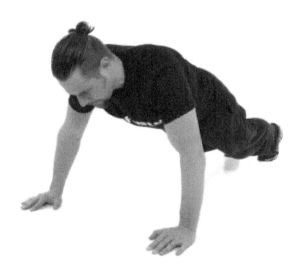

# Military bursts (P)

## Stage 2

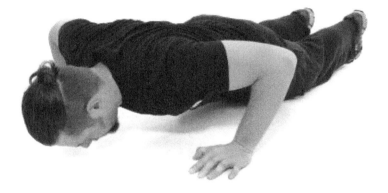

# Military bursts (P)

## Stage 3

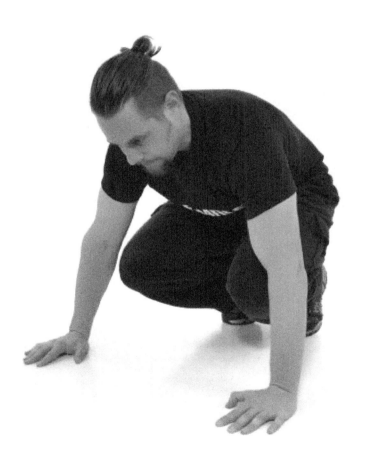

# Military bursts (P)

## Stage 4

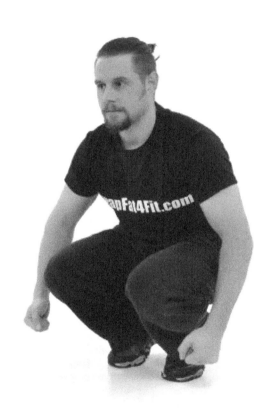

# Military bursts (P)

## Stage 5

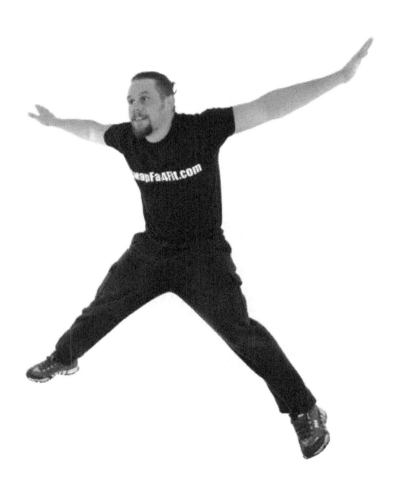

# Description Of Exercise

*(Military Bursts)*

**START POSITION:** Get in to a position on the floor so your hands are about shoulder width apart and in line with your mid/ upper chest. You should keep your back flat and take the weight of your body. Make sure that you do not dip your head. (This is the push up position)

**Movement:** Perform a single pushup, once at the top of the pushup movement, perform a squat thrust and once you are at the top of the squat thrust movement you should bring your hands off the floor and move into a position where you are squatting with your body weight resting on the balls of your feet. From this position you should explode into a star jump.

As soon as you have landed from the star jump phase, you should immediately adopt the pushup position again ready for the next rep.

This exercise should flow and you should be constantly moving throughout your exercise time slot.

# Dorsal Hyper Pulls

## Start position

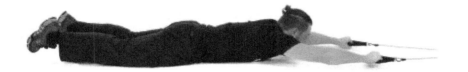

# Dorsal Hyper Pulls

## Top of movement

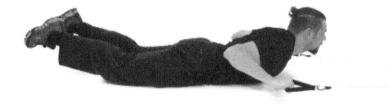

# Description Of Exercise

*(Dorsal hyper pulls)*

**START POSITION:** Thread the door attachment through your exercise band of choice and attach the stirrups to each end of this band. Secure the door attachment at the bottom of a closed door ensuring that the stirrups have equal lengths either side.

Lay face down on the floor pointing your toes so the tops of your feet are also in contact with the floor. This position should also be in front of the door that you have attached your exercise band to and at a far enough distance away that when gripping the stirrups (palms facing down), the exercise band is taught when your arms are extended out in front of you

You should keep a flat back and your head and neck should keep this alignment.

**Movement:** As you exhale you should pull your fists down towards your shoulders whilst simultaneously performing a dorsal raise.

To make this a bit more challenging and bring in your lower back muscles more, you can also try raising your feet off the floor as well.

Once at the top of the movement, you should inhale as you return to the start position.

# Close grip push ups

## Start position

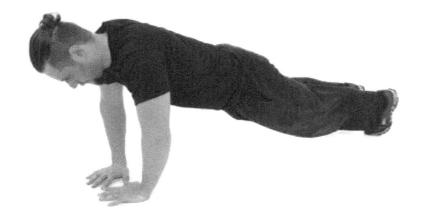

# Close grip push ups

## Top of movement

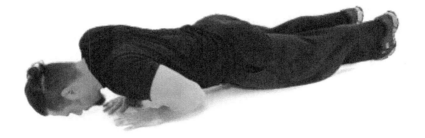

# Description Of Exercise

*(Close grip pushups)*

**START POSITION:** Get in to a position on the floor so your thumbs are touching and your hands are directly below your chest. Your elbows should be slightly bent and locked into this position. You should keep your back flat and take the weight of your body. Make sure that you do not dip your head.

**Movement:** Keep your back straight and lower your upper body towards the floor by bending your elbows and breathing in. Allow your elbows to flare out naturally to the sides of your body whilst moving to the top of the movement. Once you are at the top of this movement, as you exhale, raise your upper body back to the starting position. This completes one rep.

# More information

# More info: Door attachment

This is a variation of the door attachment that I have used on several of these exercises.

It is important when using this piece of equipment that you use it on the side of a door that opens away from you.

This way there is less chance that the door will open and the attachment will come loose.

Always make sure that this attachment is very secure before using.

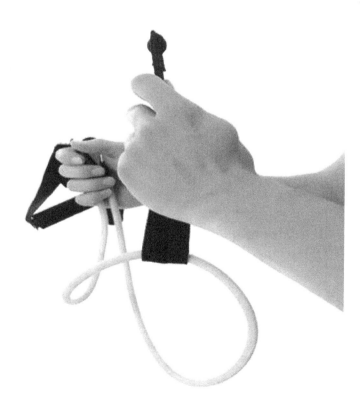

# Marathon training and distance running

———

There are many ways in which you can progress in the fitness world. There are lots of different routes that you can travel down. For instance, someone starting out may decide that they want to become more muscle bound and favor the resistance training side of fitness over the cardiovascular side.

Everyone will have a different story. Here is an excerpt from one of my other books. It is my story of becoming a long distance runner. If you do feel that you would like to take up running and work on your cardio vascular and fat burning fitness potential, why not lean from my mistakes and personal experience?

You will always get to where you want to be a whole lot quicker if you learn from someone else's mistakes.

## Excerpt from:

## "Marathon training and distance running tips"

I KNOW THERE ARE PLENTY of books out there about this type of training but I would like to share my first-hand experience of developing from a guy who couldn't run 1.5 miles in 15 minutes to a guy who could be handed a pair of running shoes and be standing confidently at the start line of a marathon in the time it took to tie those shoes up. That was all the preparation time that I needed.

Oh, and I got to a point when I could cover the same 1.5 mile distance that I was previously so bad at in 8 minutes and 22 seconds!

Let's start at the beginning;

It was summer 1999 and I had just finished my secondary school education, not being an academic and not knowing what I wanted to do with my life, I decided to enroll for a business studies class at college. It wasn't long before I realised that sitting in an office was not something that I really wanted to do. (Looking back, this was a fairly good opportunity but "you live you learn" I suppose)

Anyway, about six months in to this college education, I decided that I wanted a bit of excitement from my life and the thought of being average Joe with a regular nine to five job made me pretty depressed.

It was at this point that I ventured into the local army careers office.

"So, do you have any idea what you want to do as a job in the army?" asked the sergeant on the front desk.

I had heard a lot about airborne forces and the parachute regiment and wanted a piece of that.

"Yeah I want to look at joining the paras" I said not realizing at that time that you don't simply "join the paras"!

"Ok, let's have a chat" he replied (probably thinking "Jeez! Here's another one with absolutely no clue!")

The sergeant had a good chat with me, and concluded that I should look at getting a trade in the Royal Engineers and I could then volunteer for Para training at a later date. This way I would have a trade, be on higher pay and also get to jump out of planes and serve with airborne forces.

To go down this path however, I would need to pass the aptitude test at a higher level. I took this aptitude test 4 times with a 6 week gap between tests before the Sergeant just gave me a pass. (I actually think I failed the fourth time as well but he just fixed my score. It was good to see someone give me a chance)

So that was me going to the next stage of the army selection process. And this was the Fitness testing stage!

These fitness tests were over a long weekend where all potential recruits are taken to an army training center and tested on attitude, strength, endurance and checked if they were medically fit.

As I was into weight training at the time, I did well with the strength tests but on the last day there is a mile and a half run that must be completed in something like 15 minutes. This is very achievable and you could probably do this at a fast paced walk.

This circuit is led by a PTI who is the pace maker. If you stick with this guy, you will pass. Simple!

There were about 20 guys on this stage of the selection process with me and we all started at a steady jog close to the PTI.

At about a minute in to the test, my breathing was all over the place, my lower back was giving me pain and I started to get a stitch. I must have looked like I was at the final few miles of a marathon!

I remember the PTI turning to me and shouting;

"What's up Atkinson? You got a sucking chest wound?" Before laughing and leaving me to drop back behind the whole squad.

When I eventually crossed the finish line I gave my name to one of the corporals and he noted my time down. Needless to say this was a big fat fail and if I did want to join the army, I would have to start some kind of running programme.

Back at the careers office, the same sergeant that I had originally spoken to gave me a fitness plan to follow so I could try again in six months' time.

So getting into the army wasn't as easy as I had first thought and I was glad that I had been put on the "Trade path" rather than the "parachute regiment path" at this point.

College was still in the picture and I would get up an hour earlier each morning and run around a two mile circuit that I had planned out. At first this took 25 minutes and within a few weeks it was down to seventeen minutes. Sorted!

The time came for the next selection process and I flew through it, sticking with the PTI and being amongst the first to cross the finish line on the final mile and a half test.

I finally joined the army in 2001 so this had taken me the best part of two years!

# One Last Thing....

———

I would like to take this opportunity to send you a sincere thank you for purchasing this book. It really means a lot to me that you chose this over all of the other competition.

I would also like to let you know that this was Self-published. This means that I have had no help with promotion or financial backing in the writing, editing, design and publishing process of this book.

I strongly believe that this is a very good guide and I would like to get it into the hands of as many people in need of real weight loss and fitness help as possible.

Therefore I would be delighted if you would mention this to your friends if you think that they will benefit from it. Facebook it, tweet it, blog it! ☺

Many thanks, good luck and I look forward to hearing from you!

All the very best

Jim

Visit my blog for more great advice on diet, training, healthy recipes, motivation and more

www.jimshealthandmuscle.com[1]

Please also "Like" and get regular updates on my facebook page www.facebook.com/jimshealthandmuscle[2]

And Follow on Twitter

@jimshm

---

1. http://www.jimshealthandmuscle.com/

2. http://www.facebook.com/jimshealthandmuscle